FOOD AND EXERCISE JOURNAL

NEVER GIVE UP

Emma
Raine
Journals

Cover and page design by Cool Journals Studios - Copyright 2014

ISBN-13: 978-1495382949 ISBN-10: 149538294X

Month	Day			Daily Log		
Mon	Tue	Wed	Thur	Fri	Sat	Sun

Sleep   1 2 3 4 5 6 7 8 9 10
Stress   1 2 3 4 5 6 7 8 9 10
Exertion   1 2 3 4 5 6 7 8 9 10
Energy Level   1 2 3 4 5 6 7 8 9 10

Glasses of Water

Breakfast   CALORIES

Lunch   CALORIES

Dinner   CALORIES

W O D
workout of the day

Warmup

Workout

Recovery

Mon	Tue	Wed	Thur	Fri	Sat	Sun

Sleep　　　1 2 3 4 5 6 7 8 9 10

Stress　　1 2 3 4 5 6 7 8 9 10

Exertion　1 2 3 4 5 6 7 8 9 10

Energy Level　1 2 3 4 5 6 7 8 9 10

Glasses of Water

Breakfast　CALORIES

3 Sausage Links

2 eggs

Lunch　CALORIES

Dinner　CALORIES

W O D
workout of the day

Warmup

Workout

Recovery

Mon   Tue   Wed   Thur   Fri   Sat   Sun

S l e e p	1 2 3 4 5 6 7 8 9 10
S t r e s s	1 2 3 4 5 6 7 8 9 10
E x e r t i o n	1 2 3 4 5 6 7 8 9 10
Energy Level	1 2 3 4 5 6 7 8 9 10

Glasses of Water

Breakfast   CALORIES

_____

_____

_____

_____

_____

_____

_____

_____

Lunch   CALORIES

Dinner   CALORIES

W O D
workout of the day

Warmup _____

Workout _____

_____

_____

_____

_____

_____

Recovery _____

Month		Day			Daily Log		
Mon	Tue	Wed	Thur	Fri	Sat	Sun	

Sleep   1 2 3 4 5 6 7 8 9 10

Stress   1 2 3 4 5 6 7 8 9 10

Exertion   1 2 3 4 5 6 7 8 9 10

Energy Level   1 2 3 4 5 6 7 8 9 10

Glasses of Water

Breakfast   CALORIE

Lunch   CALORIES

Dinner   CALORIE

W O D
workout of the day

Warmup

Workout

Recovery

Month	Day				Daily Log		
Mon	Tue	Wed	Thur	Fri	Sat	Sun	

Sleep   1 2 3 4 5 6 7 8 9 10

Stress   1 2 3 4 5 6 7 8 9 10

Exertion   1 2 3 4 5 6 7 8 9 10

Energy Level   1 2 3 4 5 6 7 8 9 10

Glasses of Water

Breakfast   CALORIES

Lunch   CALORIES

Dinner   CALORIES

W O D
workout of the day

Warmup

Workout

Recovery

| Mon | Tue | Wed | Thur | Fri | Sat | Sun |

Sleep   1 2 3 4 5 6 7 8 9 10

Stress   1 2 3 4 5 6 7 8 9 10

Exertion   1 2 3 4 5 6 7 8 9 10

Energy Level   1 2 3 4 5 6 7 8 9 10

Glasses of Water

| Breakfast | CALORIE |

Lunch   CALORIES

Dinner   CALORIE

W O D
workout of the day

Warmup

Workout

Recovery

Mon   Tue   Wed   Thur   Fri   Sat   Sun

Sleep	1 2 3 4 5 6 7 8 9 10	**Breakfast** CALORIES
Stress	1 2 3 4 5 6 7 8 9 10	
Exertion	1 2 3 4 5 6 7 8 9 10	
Energy Level	1 2 3 4 5 6 7 8 9 10	

Glasses of Water

Lunch   CALORIES

Dinner   CALORIES

W O D
workout of the day

Warmup

Workout

Recovery

| Mon | Tue | Wed | Thur | Fri | Sat | Sun |

S l e e p   1 2 3 4 5 6 7 8 9 10

S t r e s s   1 2 3 4 5 6 7 8 9 10

E x e r t i o n   1 2 3 4 5 6 7 8 9 10

Energy Level   1 2 3 4 5 6 7 8 9 10

Glasses of Water

Breakfast   CALORIES

_____

_____

_____

_____

_____

_____

_____

| Lunch | CALORIES | Dinner | CALORIES |

_____   _____

_____   _____

_____   _____

_____   _____

_____   _____

_____   _____

W O D
workout of the day

Warmup _____

Workout _____

_____

_____

_____

_____

Recovery _____

Month	Day			Daily Log		
Mon	Tue	Wed	Thur	Fri	Sat	Sun

Sleep   1 2 3 4 5 6 7 8 9 10

Stress   1 2 3 4 5 6 7 8 9 10

Exertion   1 2 3 4 5 6 7 8 9 10

Energy Level   1 2 3 4 5 6 7 8 9 10

Glasses of Water

Breakfast   CALORIES

Lunch   CALORIES

Dinner   CALORIES

W O D
workout of the day

Warmup

Workout

Recovery

Mon	Tue	Wed	Thur	Fri	Sat	Sun

Sleep   1 2 3 4 5 6 7 8 9 10

Stress   1 2 3 4 5 6 7 8 9 10

Exertion   1 2 3 4 5 6 7 8 9 10

Energy Level 1 2 3 4 5 6 7 8 9 10

Glasses of Water

Breakfast   CALORIE

_____

_____

_____

_____

_____

_____

_____

_____

Lunch	CALORIES		Dinner	CALORIE

_____

_____

_____

_____

_____

_____

W O D
workout of the day

Warmup _____

Workout _____

_____

_____

_____

_____

Recovery _____

| Mon | Tue | Wed | Thur | Fri | Sat | Sun |

Sleep   1 2 3 4 5 6 7 8 9 10
Stress   1 2 3 4 5 6 7 8 9 10
Exertion   1 2 3 4 5 6 7 8 9 10
Energy Level   1 2 3 4 5 6 7 8 9 10

Glasses of Water

Breakfast   CALORIES

_____
_____
_____
_____
_____
_____

Lunch   CALORIES

_____
_____
_____
_____
_____
_____

Dinner   CALORIES

_____
_____
_____
_____
_____
_____

W O D
workout of the day

Warmup _____

Workout _____
_____
_____
_____
_____
_____

Recovery _____

| Mon | Tue | Wed | Thur | Fri | Sat | Sun |

Sleep   1 2 3 4 5 6 7 8 9 10
Stress   1 2 3 4 5 6 7 8 9 10
Exertion   1 2 3 4 5 6 7 8 9 10
Energy Level 1 2 3 4 5 6 7 8 9 10

Glasses of Water

Breakfast   CALORIE

_____
_____
_____
_____
_____
_____
_____

Lunch   CALORIES

_____
_____
_____
_____
_____
_____

Dinner   CALORIE

_____
_____
_____
_____
_____
_____

W O D
workout of the day

Warmup _____

Workout _____
_____
_____
_____
_____

Recovery _____

Month	Day			Daily Log		

Mon   Tue   Wed   Thur   Fri   Sat   Sun

Sleep   1 2 3 4 5 6 7 8 9 10
Stress   1 2 3 4 5 6 7 8 9 10
Exertion   1 2 3 4 5 6 7 8 9 10
Energy Level   1 2 3 4 5 6 7 8 9 10

Breakfast	CALORIES

Glasses of Water

Lunch	CALORIES	Dinner	CALORIES

W O D
workout of the day

Warmup _____

Workout _____

_____

_____

_____

_____

Recovery _____

Mon	Tue	Wed	Thur	Fri	Sat	Sun

Sleep   1 2 3 4 5 6 7 8 9 10

Stress   1 2 3 4 5 6 7 8 9 10

Exertion   1 2 3 4 5 6 7 8 9 10

Energy Level   1 2 3 4 5 6 7 8 9 10

Glasses of Water

Breakfast   CALORIES

Lunch   CALORIES

Dinner   CALORIES

W O D
workout of the day

Warmup

Workout

Recovery

| Mon | Tue | Wed | Thur | Fri | Sat | Sun |

Sleep   1 2 3 4 5 6 7 8 9 10
Stress   1 2 3 4 5 6 7 8 9 10
Exertion   1 2 3 4 5 6 7 8 9 10
Energy Level   1 2 3 4 5 6 7 8 9 10

Glasses of Water

Breakfast   CALORIES

_____
_____
_____
_____
_____
_____
_____

Lunch   CALORIES

_____
_____
_____
_____
_____
_____
_____

Dinner   CALORIES

_____
_____
_____
_____
_____
_____
_____

W O D
workout of the day

Warmup _____

Workout _____
_____
_____
_____
_____
_____

Recovery _____

Mon　　Tue　　Wed　　Thur　　Fri　　Sat　　Sun

Sleep　　　　1 2 3 4 5 6 7 8 9 10　　Breakfast　　CALORIE

Stress　　　1 2 3 4 5 6 7 8 9 10

Exertion　　1 2 3 4 5 6 7 8 9 10 _____

Energy Level　1 2 3 4 5 6 7 8 9 10 _____

Glasses of Water

_____

_____

_____

_____

_____

_____

Lunch　　CALORIES　　　　Dinner　　CALORIE

W O D
workout of the day

Warmup _____

Workout _____

_____

_____

_____

_____

Recovery _____

Mon	Tue	Wed	Thur	Fri	Sat	Sun

Sleep	1 2 3 4 5 6 7 8 9 10	
Stress	1 2 3 4 5 6 7 8 9 10	
Exertion	1 2 3 4 5 6 7 8 9 10	
Energy Level	1 2 3 4 5 6 7 8 9 10	

Glasses of Water

Breakfast CALORIES

Lunch CALORIES

Dinner CALORIES

W O D
workout of the day

Warmup

Workout

Recovery

Mon	Tue	Wed	Thur	Fri	Sat	Sun

Sleep   1 2 3 4 5 6 7 8 9 10

Stress   1 2 3 4 5 6 7 8 9 10

Exertion   1 2 3 4 5 6 7 8 9 10

Energy Level 1 2 3 4 5 6 7 8 9 10

Glasses of Water

Breakfast   CALORIE

_____

_____

_____

_____

_____

_____

_____

Lunch CALORIES	Dinner CALORIE
_____	_____
_____	_____
_____	_____
_____	_____
_____	_____
_____	_____
_____	_____

W O D
workout of the day

Warmup _____

Workout _____

_____

_____

_____

_____

Recovery _____

Mon   Tue   Wed   Thur   Fri   Sat   Sun

S l e e p   1 2 3 4 5 6 7 8 9 10
S t r e s s   1 2 3 4 5 6 7 8 9 10
E x e r t i o n   1 2 3 4 5 6 7 8 9 10
Energy Level   1 2 3 4 5 6 7 8 9 10

Glasses of Water

Breakfast   CALORIES

Lunch   CALORIES

Dinner   CALORIES

W   O   D
workout of the day

Warmup

Workout

Recovery

Month	Day				Daily Log	
Mon	Tue	Wed	Thur	Fri	Sat	Sun

Sleep   1 2 3 4 5 6 7 8 9 10

Stress   1 2 3 4 5 6 7 8 9 10

Exertion   1 2 3 4 5 6 7 8 9 10

Energy Level   1 2 3 4 5 6 7 8 9 10

Glasses of Water

Breakfast · CALORIES

Lunch · CALORIES

Dinner · CALORIES

W O D
workout of the day

Warmup

Workout

Recovery

Month	Day				Daily Log		
Mon	Tue	Wed	Thur	Fri	Sat	Sun	

Sleep   1 2 3 4 5 6 7 8 9 10

Stress   1 2 3 4 5 6 7 8 9 10

Exertion   1 2 3 4 5 6 7 8 9 10

Energy Level 1 2 3 4 5 6 7 8 9 10

Glasses of Water

Breakfast — CALORIES

Lunch — CALORIES

Dinner — CALORIES

W O D
workout of the day

Warmup _____

Workout _____

Recovery _____

Mon	Tue	Wed	Thur	Fri	Sat	Sun

Sleep   1 2 3 4 5 6 7 8 9 10   **Breakfast**   CALORIES
Stress   1 2 3 4 5 6 7 8 9 10
Exertion   1 2 3 4 5 6 7 8 9 10   _____
Energy Level   1 2 3 4 5 6 7 8 9 10   _____

Glasses of Water

_____

_____

_____

_____

_____

_____

Lunch	CALORIES		**Dinner**	CALORIES

W O D
workout of the day

Warmup _____

Workout _____

_____

_____

_____

Recovery _____

| Mon | Tue | Wed | Thur | Fri | Sat | Sun |

Sleep   1 2 3 4 5 6 7 8 9 10

Stress   1 2 3 4 5 6 7 8 9 10

Exertion   1 2 3 4 5 6 7 8 9 10

Energy Level   1 2 3 4 5 6 7 8 9 10

Glasses of Water

Breakfast   CALORIES

Lunch   CALORIES

Dinner   CALORIES

W O D
workout of the day

Warmup

Workout

Recovery

Daily Log

Mon	Tue	Wed	Thur	Fri	Sat	Sun

S l e e p	1 2 3 4 5 6 7 8 9 10	
S t r e s s	1 2 3 4 5 6 7 8 9 10	
E x e r t i o n	1 2 3 4 5 6 7 8 9 10	
Energy Level	1 2 3 4 5 6 7 8 9 10	

Glasses of Water

Breakfast   CALORIE

_____

_____

_____

_____

_____

_____

_____

_____

Lunch CALORIES	Dinner CALORIE
_____	_____
_____	_____
_____	_____
_____	_____
_____	_____
_____	_____
_____	_____

W O D
workout of the day

Warmup _____

Workout _____

_____

_____

_____

_____

Recovery _____

Month	Day			Daily Log		

Mon	Tue	Wed	Thur	Fri	Sat	Sun

Sleep   1 2 3 4 5 6 7 8 9 10

Stress   1 2 3 4 5 6 7 8 9 10

Exertion   1 2 3 4 5 6 7 8 9 10

Energy Level   1 2 3 4 5 6 7 8 9 10

Glasses of Water

Breakfast   CALORIES

Lunch   CALORIES

Dinner   CALORIES

W O D
workout of the day

Warmup

Workout

Recovery

Month	Day				Daily Log	
Mon	Tue	Wed	Thur	Fri	Sat	Sun

S l e e p	1 2 3 4 5 6 7 8 9 10	
S t r e s s	1 2 3 4 5 6 7 8 9 10	
Exertion	1 2 3 4 5 6 7 8 9 10	
Energy Level	1 2 3 4 5 6 7 8 9 10	

Breakfast CALORIES

_____
_____
_____
_____
_____
_____
_____

Glasses of Water

Lunch	CALORIES
_____	
_____	
_____	
_____	
_____	
_____	

Dinner	CALORIES
_____	
_____	
_____	
_____	
_____	
_____	

W O D
workout of the day

Warmup _____

Workout _____

_____

_____

_____

_____

Recovery _____

Month	Day				Daily Log		
Mon	Tue	Wed	Thur	Fri	Sat	Sun	

Sleep   1 2 3 4 5 6 7 8 9 10
Stress   1 2 3 4 5 6 7 8 9 10
Exertion   1 2 3 4 5 6 7 8 9 10
Energy Level   1 2 3 4 5 6 7 8 9 10

Glasses of Water

Breakfast   CALORIES

_____
_____
_____
_____
_____
_____
_____

Lunch   CALORIES

_____
_____
_____
_____
_____
_____
_____

Dinner   CALORIES

_____
_____
_____
_____
_____
_____
_____

W O D
workout of the day

Warmup _____

Workout _____
_____
_____
_____
_____
_____

Recovery _____

Month		Day			Daily Log		
Mon	Tue	Wed	Thur	Fri	Sat	Sun

Sleep   1 2 3 4 5 6 7 8 9 10

Stress   1 2 3 4 5 6 7 8 9 10

Exertion   1 2 3 4 5 6 7 8 9 10

Energy Level 1 2 3 4 5 6 7 8 9 10

Glasses of Water

Breakfast   CALORIES

_____

_____

_____

_____

_____

_____

_____

Lunch	CALORIES	Dinner	CALORIES

_____

_____

_____

_____

_____

_____

W   O   D
workout of the day

Warmup _____

Workout _____

_____

_____

_____

_____

Recovery _____

Month		Day			Daily Log		
Mon	Tue	Wed	Thur	Fri	Sat	Sun	

			Breakfast	CALORIES
Sleep	1 2 3 4 5 6 7 8 9 10			
Stress	1 2 3 4 5 6 7 8 9 10			
Exertion	1 2 3 4 5 6 7 8 9 10			
Energy Level	1 2 3 4 5 6 7 8 9 10			

Glasses of Water

Lunch   CALORIES

Dinner   CALORIES

W O D
workout of the day

Warmup

Workout

Recovery

Mon	Tue	Wed	Thur	Fri	Sat	Sun

Sleep   1 2 3 4 5 6 7 8 9 10
Stress   1 2 3 4 5 6 7 8 9 10
Exertion   1 2 3 4 5 6 7 8 9 10
Energy Level 1 2 3 4 5 6 7 8 9 10

Glasses of Water

Breakfast   CALORIE

Lunch   CALORIES

Dinner   CALORIE

W O D
workout of the day

Warmup

Workout

Recovery

Month	Day					Daily Log
Mon	Tue	Wed	Thur	Fri	Sat	Sun

Sleep   1 2 3 4 5 6 7 8 9 10

Stress   1 2 3 4 5 6 7 8 9 10

Exertion   1 2 3 4 5 6 7 8 9 10

Energy Level   1 2 3 4 5 6 7 8 9 10

Glasses of Water

Breakfast   CALORIES

Lunch   CALORIES

Dinner   CALORIES

W O D
workout of the day

Warmup

Workout

Recovery

| Mon | Tue | Wed | Thur | Fri | Sat | Sun |

Sleep   1 2 3 4 5 6 7 8 9 10
Stress   1 2 3 4 5 6 7 8 9 10
Exertion   1 2 3 4 5 6 7 8 9 10
Energy Level   1 2 3 4 5 6 7 8 9 10

Glasses of Water

Breakfast   CALORIES

Lunch   CALORIES

Dinner   CALORIES

W O D
workout of the day

Warmup

Workout

Recovery

| Mon | Tue | Wed | Thur | Fri | Sat | Sun |

Sleep   1 2 3 4 5 6 7 8 9 10
Stress   1 2 3 4 5 6 7 8 9 10
Exertion   1 2 3 4 5 6 7 8 9 10
Energy Level   1 2 3 4 5 6 7 8 9 10

Glasses of Water

Breakfast   CALORIES

_____

_____

_____

_____

_____

_____

Lunch   CALORIES

_____

_____

_____

_____

_____

_____

Dinner   CALORIES

_____

_____

_____

_____

_____

_____

W O D
workout of the day

Warmup _____

Workout _____

_____

_____

_____

_____

Recovery _____

Month	Day				Daily Log		
Mon	Tue	Wed	Thur	Fri	Sat	Sun	

Sleep   1 2 3 4 5 6 7 8 9 10
Stress   1 2 3 4 5 6 7 8 9 10
Exertion   1 2 3 4 5 6 7 8 9 10
Energy Level   1 2 3 4 5 6 7 8 9 10

Glasses of Water

Breakfast   CALORIES

_____
_____
_____
_____
_____
_____
_____

Lunch   CALORIES

_____
_____
_____
_____
_____
_____

Dinner   CALORIES

_____
_____
_____
_____
_____
_____

W O D
workout of the day

Warmup _____
Workout _____
_____
_____
_____
_____

Recovery _____

| Mon | Tue | Wed | Thur | Fri | Sat | Sun |

S l e e p   1 2 3 4 5 6 7 8 9 10

S t r e s s   1 2 3 4 5 6 7 8 9 10

E x e r t i o n   1 2 3 4 5 6 7 8 9 10

Energy Level   1 2 3 4 5 6 7 8 9 10

Glasses of Water

Breakfast   CALORIES

_____

_____

_____

_____

_____

_____

_____

| Lunch | CALORIES | Dinner | CALORIES |

W O D
workout of the day

Warmup _____

Workout _____

_____

_____

_____

Recovery _____

Month	Day				Daily Log		
Mon	Tue	Wed	Thur	Fri	Sat	Sun

Sleep   1 2 3 4 5 6 7 8 9 10
Stress   1 2 3 4 5 6 7 8 9 10
Exertion   1 2 3 4 5 6 7 8 9 10
Energy Level   1 2 3 4 5 6 7 8 9 10

Glasses of Water

Breakfast   CALORIES

_____
_____
_____
_____
_____
_____
_____

Lunch   CALORIES

_____
_____
_____
_____
_____
_____

Dinner   CALORIES

_____
_____
_____
_____
_____
_____

W O D
workout of the day

Warmup _____

Workout _____
_____
_____
_____
_____

Recovery _____

Month	Day			Daily Log		
Mon	Tue	Wed	Thur	Fri	Sat	Sun

Sleep   1 2 3 4 5 6 7 8 9 10
Stress   1 2 3 4 5 6 7 8 9 10
Exertion   1 2 3 4 5 6 7 8 9 10
Energy Level 1 2 3 4 5 6 7 8 9 10

Glasses of Water

Breakfast   CALORIES

_____

_____

_____

_____

_____

_____

Lunch   CALORIES

_____

_____

_____

_____

_____

_____

_____

Dinner   CALORIES

_____

_____

_____

_____

_____

_____

_____

W O D
workout of the day

Warmup _____

Workout _____

_____

_____

_____

_____

Recovery _____

Mon	Tue	Wed	Thur	Fri	Sat	Sun

Sleep   1 2 3 4 5 6 7 8 9 10

Stress   1 2 3 4 5 6 7 8 9 10

Exertion   1 2 3 4 5 6 7 8 9 10

Energy Level 1 2 3 4 5 6 7 8 9 10

Glasses of Water

Breakfast — CALORIES

_____

_____

_____

_____

_____

_____

_____

_____

Lunch — CALORIES

_____

_____

_____

_____

_____

_____

Dinner — CALORIES

_____

_____

_____

_____

_____

_____

W O D
workout of the day

Warmup _____

Workout _____

_____

_____

_____

_____

Recovery _____

Mon	Tue	Wed	Thur	Fri	Sat	Sun

Sleep   1 2 3 4 5 6 7 8 9 10

Stress   1 2 3 4 5 6 7 8 9 10

Exertion   1 2 3 4 5 6 7 8 9 10

Energy Level 1 2 3 4 5 6 7 8 9 10

Glasses of Water

Breakfast   CALORIES

Lunch   CALORIES

Dinner   CALORIES

W O D
workout of the day

Warmup

Workout

Recovery

Mon   Tue   Wed   Thur   Fri   Sat   Sun

Sleep   1 2 3 4 5 6 7 8 9 10
Stress   1 2 3 4 5 6 7 8 9 10
Exertion   1 2 3 4 5 6 7 8 9 10
Energy Level   1 2 3 4 5 6 7 8 9 10

Glasses of Water

Breakfast   CALORIES

Lunch   CALORIES

Dinner   CALORIES

W O D
workout of the day

Warmup

Workout

Recovery

Mon   Tue   Wed   Thur   Fri   Sat   Sun

Sleep   1 2 3 4 5 6 7 8 9 10   Breakfast   CALORIES
Stress   1 2 3 4 5 6 7 8 9 10
Exertion   1 2 3 4 5 6 7 8 9 10   _____
Energy Level   1 2 3 4 5 6 7 8 9 10   _____

Glasses of Water

_____

_____

_____

_____

_____

Lunch	CALORIES	Dinner	CALORIES

W O D
workout of the day

Warmup _____

Workout _____

_____

_____

_____

Recovery _____

| Mon | Tue | Wed | Thur | Fri | Sat | Sun |

Sleep	1 2 3 4 5 6 7 8 9 10
Stress	1 2 3 4 5 6 7 8 9 10
Exertion	1 2 3 4 5 6 7 8 9 10
Energy Level	1 2 3 4 5 6 7 8 9 10

Glasses of Water

Breakfast CALORIES

Lunch CALORIES

Dinner CALORIES

W O D
workout of the day

Warmup

Workout

Recovery

Sleep   1 2 3 4 5 6 7 8 9 10
Stress   1 2 3 4 5 6 7 8 9 10
Exertion   1 2 3 4 5 6 7 8 9 10
Energy Level   1 2 3 4 5 6 7 8 9 10

Glasses of Water

Breakfast   CALORIES

_____ _____
_____ _____
_____ _____
_____ _____
_____ _____
_____ _____
_____ _____

Lunch   CALORIES

_____ _____
_____ _____
_____ _____
_____ _____
_____ _____
_____ _____

Dinner   CALORIES

_____ _____
_____ _____
_____ _____
_____ _____
_____ _____
_____ _____

W O D
workout of the day

Warmup _____

Workout _____
_____
_____
_____
_____
_____

Recovery _____

| Mon | Tue | Wed | Thur | Fri | Sat | Sun |

Sleep   1 2 3 4 5 6 7 8 9 10

Stress   1 2 3 4 5 6 7 8 9 10

Exertion   1 2 3 4 5 6 7 8 9 10

Energy Level   1 2 3 4 5 6 7 8 9 10

Glasses of Water

Breakfast   CALORIES

Lunch   CALORIES

Dinner   CALORIES

W O D
workout of the day

Warmup

Workout

Recovery

| Mon | Tue | Wed | Thur | Fri | Sat | Sun |

Sleep   1 2 3 4 5 6 7 8 9 10

Stress   1 2 3 4 5 6 7 8 9 10

Exertion   1 2 3 4 5 6 7 8 9 10

Energy Level   1 2 3 4 5 6 7 8 9 10

Glasses of Water

Breakfast   CALORIES

_____

_____

_____

_____

_____

_____

_____

Lunch   CALORIES

_____

_____

_____

_____

_____

_____

Dinner   CALORIES

_____

_____

_____

_____

_____

_____

W O D
workout of the day

Warmup _____

Workout _____

_____

_____

_____

_____

_____

Recovery _____

| Mon | Tue | Wed | Thur | Fri | Sat | Sun |

Sleep   1 2 3 4 5 6 7 8 9 10
Stress   1 2 3 4 5 6 7 8 9 10
Exertion   1 2 3 4 5 6 7 8 9 10
Energy Level   1 2 3 4 5 6 7 8 9 10

Glasses of Water

Breakfast   CALORIES

_____

_____

_____

_____

_____

_____

_____

_____

Lunch CALORIES	Dinner CALORIES
_____	_____
_____	_____
_____	_____
_____	_____
_____	_____
_____	_____

W O D
workout of the day

Warmup _____

Workout _____

_____

_____

_____

Recovery _____

Month		Day			Daily Log		
Mon	Tue	Wed	Thur	Fri	Sat	Sun

Sleep   1 2 3 4 5 6 7 8 9 10
Stress   1 2 3 4 5 6 7 8 9 10
Exertion   1 2 3 4 5 6 7 8 9 10
Energy Level 1 2 3 4 5 6 7 8 9 10

Glasses of Water

Breakfast	CALORIES

Lunch	CALORIES		Dinner	CALORIES

W O D
workout of the day

Warmup

Workout

Recovery

| Mon | Tue | Wed | Thur | Fri | Sat | Sun |

S l e e p   1 2 3 4 5 6 7 8 9 10
S t r e s s   1 2 3 4 5 6 7 8 9 10
E x e r t i o n 1 2 3 4 5 6 7 8 9 10
Energy Level   1 2 3 4 5 6 7 8 9 10

Glasses of Water

Breakfast   CALORIES

_____
_____
_____
_____
_____
_____
_____

Lunch   CALORIES

_____
_____
_____
_____
_____
_____

Dinner   CALORIES

_____
_____
_____
_____
_____
_____

W O D
workout of the day

Warmup _____

Workout _____

_____
_____
_____
_____

Recovery _____

Mon   Tue   Wed   Thur   Fri   Sat   Sun

S l e e p   1 2 3 4 5 6 7 8 9 10

S t r e s s   1 2 3 4 5 6 7 8 9 10

Exertion   1 2 3 4 5 6 7 8 9 10

Energy Level   1 2 3 4 5 6 7 8 9 10

Glasses of Water

Breakfast   CALORIES

_____   _____

_____   _____

_____   _____

_____   _____

_____   _____

_____   _____

Lunch   CALORIES

Dinner   CALORIES

W O D
workout of the day

Warmup _____

Workout _____

_____

_____

_____

_____

Recovery _____

| Mon | Tue | Wed | Thur | Fri | Sat | Sun |

Sleep   1 2 3 4 5 6 7 8 9 10

Stress   1 2 3 4 5 6 7 8 9 10

Exertion   1 2 3 4 5 6 7 8 9 10

Energy Level   1 2 3 4 5 6 7 8 9 10

Glasses of Water

Breakfast   CALORIES

Lunch   CALORIES

Dinner   CALORIES

W O D
workout of the day

Warmup

Workout

Recovery

Mon   Tue   Wed   Thur   Fri   Sat   Sun

S l e e p   1 2 3 4 5 6 7 8 9 10   Breakfast   CALORIES
S t r e s s   1 2 3 4 5 6 7 8 9 10
E x e r t i o n   1 2 3 4 5 6 7 8 9 10
Energy Level   1 2 3 4 5 6 7 8 9 10

Glasses of Water

Lunch   CALORIES   Dinner   CALORIES

W O D
workout of the day

Warmup

Workout

Recovery

| Mon | Tue | Wed | Thur | Fri | Sat | Sun |

Sleep   1 2 3 4 5 6 7 8 9 10
Stress   1 2 3 4 5 6 7 8 9 10
Exertion 1 2 3 4 5 6 7 8 9 10
Energy Level 1 2 3 4 5 6 7 8 9 10

Glasses of Water

Breakfast · CALORIES

_____
_____
_____
_____
_____
_____
_____
_____

Lunch · CALORIES

_____
_____
_____
_____
_____
_____

Dinner · CALORIES

_____
_____
_____
_____
_____
_____

W O D
workout of the day

Warmup _____

Workout _____
_____
_____
_____
_____
_____

Recovery _____

| Mon | Tue | Wed | Thur | Fri | Sat | Sun |

Sleep   1 2 3 4 5 6 7 8 9 10

Stress   1 2 3 4 5 6 7 8 9 10

Exertion   1 2 3 4 5 6 7 8 9 10

Energy Level   1 2 3 4 5 6 7 8 9 10

Glasses of Water

Breakfast   CALORIES

_____

_____

_____

_____

_____

_____

_____

Lunch   CALORIES

_____

_____

_____

_____

_____

_____

Dinner   CALORIES

_____

_____

_____

_____

_____

_____

W O D
workout of the day

Warmup _____

Workout _____

_____

_____

_____

_____

Recovery _____

| Mon | Tue | Wed | Thur | Fri | Sat | Sun |

S l e e p   1 2 3 4 5 6 7 8 9 10

S t r e s s   1 2 3 4 5 6 7 8 9 10

Exertion   1 2 3 4 5 6 7 8 9 10

Energy Level   1 2 3 4 5 6 7 8 9 10

Breakfast   CALORIES

Glasses of Water

Lunch   CALORIES

Dinner   CALORIES

W O D
workout of the day

Warmup

Workout

Recovery

Month	Day				Daily Log	
Mon	Tue	Wed	Thur	Fri	Sat	Sun

Sleep   1 2 3 4 5 6 7 8 9 10
Stress   1 2 3 4 5 6 7 8 9 10
Exertion   1 2 3 4 5 6 7 8 9 10
Energy Level 1 2 3 4 5 6 7 8 9 10

Glasses of Water

Breakfast   CALORIES

_____
_____
_____
_____
_____
_____
_____

Lunch   CALORIES

_____
_____
_____
_____
_____
_____

Dinner   CALORIES

_____
_____
_____
_____
_____
_____

W O D
workout of the day

Warmup _____

Workout _____

_____
_____
_____
_____

Recovery _____

| Mon | Tue | Wed | Thur | Fri | Sat | Sun |

Sleep   1 2 3 4 5 6 7 8 9 10
Stress   1 2 3 4 5 6 7 8 9 10
Exertion   1 2 3 4 5 6 7 8 9 10
Energy Level   1 2 3 4 5 6 7 8 9 10

Glasses of Water

Breakfast   CALORIES
_____
_____
_____
_____
_____
_____
_____

Lunch   CALORIES

_____
_____
_____
_____
_____
_____

Dinner   CALORIES

_____
_____
_____
_____
_____
_____

W O D
workout of the day

Warmup _____

Workout _____
_____
_____
_____
_____

Recovery _____

Month	Day	Daily Log

Mon   Tue   Wed   Thur   Fri   Sat   Sun

Sleep   1 2 3 4 5 6 7 8 9 10
Stress   1 2 3 4 5 6 7 8 9 10
Exertion   1 2 3 4 5 6 7 8 9 10
Energy Level   1 2 3 4 5 6 7 8 9 10

Glasses of Water

Breakfast   CALORIES

_____
_____
_____
_____
_____
_____
_____

Lunch   CALORIES

_____
_____
_____
_____
_____
_____
_____

Dinner   CALORIES

_____
_____
_____
_____
_____
_____
_____

W O D
workout of the day

Warmup _____
Workout _____
_____
_____
_____
_____

Recovery _____

Daily Log

| Mon | Tue | Wed | Thur | Fri | Sat | Sun |

Sleep   1 2 3 4 5 6 7 8 9 10
Stress   1 2 3 4 5 6 7 8 9 10
Exertion   1 2 3 4 5 6 7 8 9 10
Energy Level 1 2 3 4 5 6 7 8 9 10

Glasses of Water

Breakfast   CALORIES

_____
_____
_____
_____
_____
_____
_____

Lunch   CALORIES

_____
_____
_____
_____
_____
_____

Dinner   CALORIES

_____
_____
_____
_____
_____
_____

W O D
workout of the day

Warmup _____

Workout _____
_____
_____
_____
_____

Recovery _____

Month	Day			Daily Log		
Mon	Tue	Wed	Thur	Fri	Sat	Sun

Sleep   1 2 3 4 5 6 7 8 9 10
Stress   1 2 3 4 5 6 7 8 9 10
Exertion   1 2 3 4 5 6 7 8 9 10
Energy Level 1 2 3 4 5 6 7 8 9 10

Glasses of Water

Breakfast   CALORIES

_____

_____

_____

_____

_____

_____

_____

Lunch   CALORIES

_____

_____

_____

_____

_____

_____

Dinner   CALORIES

_____

_____

_____

_____

_____

_____

W O D
workout of the day

Warmup _____

Workout _____

_____

_____

_____

_____

Recovery _____

Mon	Tue	Wed	Thur	Fri	Sat	Sun

Sleep   1 2 3 4 5 6 7 8 9 10

Stress   1 2 3 4 5 6 7 8 9 10

Exertion   1 2 3 4 5 6 7 8 9 10

Energy Level   1 2 3 4 5 6 7 8 9 10

Glasses of Water

Breakfast	CALORIES
_____	_____
_____	_____
_____	_____
_____	_____
_____	_____
_____	_____
_____	_____

Lunch	CALORIES
_____	_____
_____	_____
_____	_____
_____	_____
_____	_____
_____	_____

Dinner	CALORIES
_____	_____
_____	_____
_____	_____
_____	_____
_____	_____
_____	_____

W O D
workout of the day

Warmup _____

Workout _____

_____

_____

_____

Recovery _____

Month	Day				Daily Log		
Mon	Tue	Wed	Thur	Fri	Sat	Sun	

Sleep   1 2 3 4 5 6 7 8 9 10

Stress   1 2 3 4 5 6 7 8 9 10

Exertion   1 2 3 4 5 6 7 8 9 10

Energy Level 1 2 3 4 5 6 7 8 9 10

Glasses of Water

Breakfast   CALORIES

Lunch   CALORIES

Dinner   CALORIES

W O D
workout of the day

Warmup

Workout

Recovery

Mon	Tue	Wed	Thur	Fri	Sat	Sun

Sleep   1 2 3 4 5 6 7 8 9 10

Stress   1 2 3 4 5 6 7 8 9 10

Exertion   1 2 3 4 5 6 7 8 9 10

Energy Level   1 2 3 4 5 6 7 8 9 10

Glasses of Water

Breakfast   CALORIES

Lunch   CALORIES

Dinner   CALORIES

W O D
workout of the day

Warmup

Workout

Recovery

Daily Log

Mon   Tue   Wed   Thur   Fri   Sat   Sun

Sleep   1 2 3 4 5 6 7 8 9 10
Stress   1 2 3 4 5 6 7 8 9 10
Exertion   1 2 3 4 5 6 7 8 9 10
Energy Level   1 2 3 4 5 6 7 8 9 10

Breakfast   CALORIES

Glasses of Water

Lunch   CALORIES

Dinner   CALORIES

W O D
workout of the day

Warmup

Workout

Recovery

Mon   Tue   Wed   Thur   Fri   Sat   Sun

Sleep   1 2 3 4 5 6 7 8 9 10   Breakfast   CALORIES

Stress   1 2 3 4 5 6 7 8 9 10

Exertion   1 2 3 4 5 6 7 8 9 10

Energy Level   1 2 3 4 5 6 7 8 9 10

Glasses of Water

Lunch	CALORIES	Dinner	CALORIES

W O D
workout of the day

Warmup

Workout

Recovery

Mon	Tue	Wed	Thur	Fri	Sat	Sun

Sleep   1 2 3 4 5 6 7 8 9 10
Stress   1 2 3 4 5 6 7 8 9 10
Exertion   1 2 3 4 5 6 7 8 9 10
Energy Level   1 2 3 4 5 6 7 8 9 10

Glasses of Water

Breakfast   CALORIES

Lunch   CALORIES

Dinner   CALORIES

W O D
workout of the day

Warmup

Workout

Recovery

Mon	Tue	Wed	Thur	Fri	Sat	Sun

Sleep   1 2 3 4 5 6 7 8 9 10

Stress   1 2 3 4 5 6 7 8 9 10

Exertion   1 2 3 4 5 6 7 8 9 10

Energy Level 1 2 3 4 5 6 7 8 9 10

Glasses of Water

Breakfast   CALORIES

Lunch   CALORIES

Dinner   CALORIES

W O D
workout of the day

Warmup

Workout

Recovery

Month	Day			Daily Log		
Mon	Tue	Wed	Thur	Fri	Sat	Sun

Sleep   1 2 3 4 5 6 7 8 9 10
Stress   1 2 3 4 5 6 7 8 9 10
Exertion   1 2 3 4 5 6 7 8 9 10
Energy Level 1 2 3 4 5 6 7 8 9 10

Glasses of Water

Breakfast   CALORIES

_____

_____

_____

_____

_____

_____

_____

Lunch	CALORIES	Dinner	CALORIES

_____   _____

_____   _____

_____   _____

_____   _____

_____   _____

_____   _____

_____   _____

W O D
workout of the day

<u>Warmup</u> _____

<u>Workout</u> _____

_____

_____

_____

_____

<u>Recovery</u> _____

| Mon | Tue | Wed | Thur | Fri | Sat | Sun |

Sleep 1 2 3 4 5 6 7 8 9 10
Stress 1 2 3 4 5 6 7 8 9 10
Exertion 1 2 3 4 5 6 7 8 9 10
Energy Level 1 2 3 4 5 6 7 8 9 10

Glasses of Water

Breakfast   CALORIES

Lunch   CALORIES

Dinner   CALORIES

W O D
workout of the day

Warmup

Workout

Recovery

| Month | Day | | | | Daily Log | | |

Mon Tue Wed Thur Fri Sat Sun

Sleep   1 2 3 4 5 6 7 8 9 10
Stress   1 2 3 4 5 6 7 8 9 10
Exertion   1 2 3 4 5 6 7 8 9 10
Energy Level   1 2 3 4 5 6 7 8 9 10

Glasses of Water

| Breakfast | CALORIES |

_____
_____
_____
_____
_____
_____
_____

| Lunch | CALORIES |

_____
_____
_____
_____
_____
_____
_____

| Dinner | CALORIES |

_____
_____
_____
_____
_____
_____
_____

W O D
workout of the day

Warmup _____

Workout _____
_____
_____
_____
_____
_____

Recovery _____

Daily Log

Mon   Tue   Wed   Thur   Fri   Sat   Sun

Sleep   1 2 3 4 5 6 7 8 9 10

Stress   1 2 3 4 5 6 7 8 9 10

Exertion   1 2 3 4 5 6 7 8 9 10

Energy Level   1 2 3 4 5 6 7 8 9 10

Glasses of Water

Breakfast   CALORIES

Lunch   CALORIES

Dinner   CALORIES

W O D
workout of the day

Warmup

Workout

Recovery

Month	Day				Daily Log		
Mon	Tue	Wed	Thur	Fri	Sat	Sun

Sleep   1 2 3 4 5 6 7 8 9 10

Stress   1 2 3 4 5 6 7 8 9 10

Exertion   1 2 3 4 5 6 7 8 9 10

Energy Level   1 2 3 4 5 6 7 8 9 10

Glasses of Water

Breakfast   CALORIES

_____

_____

_____

_____

_____

_____

_____

Lunch	CALORIES	Dinner	CALORIES
_____		_____	
_____		_____	
_____		_____	
_____		_____	
_____		_____	
_____		_____	

W O D
workout of the day

Warmup _____

Workout _____

_____

_____

_____

_____

Recovery _____

| Mon | Tue | Wed | Thur | Fri | Sat | Sun |

Sleep   1 2 3 4 5 6 7 8 9 10
Stress   1 2 3 4 5 6 7 8 9 10
Exertion   1 2 3 4 5 6 7 8 9 10
Energy Level   1 2 3 4 5 6 7 8 9 10

Glasses of Water

Breakfast   CALORIES

Lunch   CALORIES

Dinner   CALORIES

W O D
workout of the day

Warmup

Workout

Recovery

Month		Day				Daily Log

Mon	Tue	Wed	Thur	Fri	Sat	Sun

Sleep   1 2 3 4 5 6 7 8 9 10

Stress   1 2 3 4 5 6 7 8 9 10

Exertion   1 2 3 4 5 6 7 8 9 10

Energy Level   1 2 3 4 5 6 7 8 9 10

Glasses of Water

Breakfast   CALORIES

Lunch   CALORIES

Dinner   CALORIES

W O D
workout of the day

Warmup

Workout

Recovery

Month	Day				Daily Log		
Mon	Tue	Wed	Thur	Fri	Sat	Sun	

Sleep 1 2 3 4 5 6 7 8 9 10

Stress 1 2 3 4 5 6 7 8 9 10

Exertion 1 2 3 4 5 6 7 8 9 10

Energy Level 1 2 3 4 5 6 7 8 9 10

Glasses of Water

Breakfast   CALORIES

_____

_____

_____

_____

_____

_____

_____

Lunch	CALORIES

Dinner	CALORIES

W O D
workout of the day

Warmup _____

Workout _____

_____

_____

_____

_____

Recovery _____

Mon   Tue   Wed   Thur   Fri   Sat   Sun

S l e e p   1 2 3 4 5 6 7 8 9 10
S t r e s s   1 2 3 4 5 6 7 8 9 10
E x e r t i o n   1 2 3 4 5 6 7 8 9 10
Energy Level   1 2 3 4 5 6 7 8 9 10

Glasses of Water

Breakfast   CALORIES

_____

_____

_____

_____

_____

_____

_____

_____

Lunch   CALORIES

_____

_____

_____

_____

_____

_____

_____

Dinner   CALORIES

_____

_____

_____

_____

_____

_____

_____

W O D
workout of the day

Warmup _____

Workout _____

_____

_____

_____

_____

Recovery _____

Mon   Tue   Wed   Thur   Fri   Sat   Sun

Sleep	1 2 3 4 5 6 7 8 9 10
Stress	1 2 3 4 5 6 7 8 9 10
Exertion	1 2 3 4 5 6 7 8 9 10
Energy Level	1 2 3 4 5 6 7 8 9 10

Glasses of Water

Breakfast   CALORIES

_____

_____

_____

_____

_____

_____

_____

Lunch   CALORIES

_____

_____

_____

_____

_____

_____

Dinner   CALORIES

_____

_____

_____

_____

_____

_____

W O D
workout of the day

Warmup _____

Workout _____

_____

_____

_____

_____

Recovery _____

Mon	Tue	Wed	Thur	Fri	Sat	Sun

Sleep   1 2 3 4 5 6 7 8 9 10

Stress   1 2 3 4 5 6 7 8 9 10

Exertion   1 2 3 4 5 6 7 8 9 10

Energy Level   1 2 3 4 5 6 7 8 9 10

Glasses of Water

Breakfast   CALORIES

Lunch   CALORIES

Dinner   CALORIES

W O D
workout of the day

<u>Warmup</u>

<u>Workout</u>

<u>Recovery</u>

| Mon | Tue | Wed | Thur | Fri | Sat | Sun |

Sleep   1 2 3 4 5 6 7 8 9 10

Stress   1 2 3 4 5 6 7 8 9 10

Exertion   1 2 3 4 5 6 7 8 9 10

Energy Level   1 2 3 4 5 6 7 8 9 10

Glasses of Water

Breakfast   CALORIES

Lunch   CALORIES

Dinner   CALORIES

W O D
workout of the day

Warmup

Workout

Recovery

Month	Day				Daily Log		
Mon	Tue	Wed	Thur	Fri	Sat	Sun

S l e e p   1 2 3 4 5 6 7 8 9 10

S t r e s s   1 2 3 4 5 6 7 8 9 10

E x e r t i o n   1 2 3 4 5 6 7 8 9 10

Energy Level   1 2 3 4 5 6 7 8 9 10

Glasses of Water

Breakfast   CALORIES

_____

_____

_____

_____

_____

_____

_____

Lunch	CALORIES

Dinner	CALORIES

W O D
workout of the day

Warmup _____

Workout _____

_____

_____

_____

_____

Recovery _____

Mon	Tue	Wed	Thur	Fri	Sat	Sun

Sleep   1 2 3 4 5 6 7 8 9 10   **Breakfast**   CALORIES

Stress   1 2 3 4 5 6 7 8 9 10

Exertion   1 2 3 4 5 6 7 8 9 10

Energy Level   1 2 3 4 5 6 7 8 9 10

Glasses of Water

Lunch	CALORIES	Dinner	CALORIES

W O D
workout of the day

__Warmup__

__Workout__

__Recovery__

Daily Log

| Mon | Tue | Wed | Thur | Fri | Sat | Sun |

Sleep   1 2 3 4 5 6 7 8 9 10
Stress   1 2 3 4 5 6 7 8 9 10
Exertion   1 2 3 4 5 6 7 8 9 10
Energy Level 1 2 3 4 5 6 7 8 9 10

Glasses of Water

Breakfast   CALORIES

_____
_____
_____
_____
_____
_____
_____

Lunch   CALORIES

_____
_____
_____
_____
_____
_____
_____

Dinner   CALORIES

_____
_____
_____
_____
_____
_____
_____

W O D
workout of the day

Warmup _____

Workout _____
_____
_____
_____
_____
_____

Recovery _____

Month		Day			Daily Log		
Mon	Tue	Wed	Thur	Fri	Sat	Sun	

Sleep   1 2 3 4 5 6 7 8 9 10
Stress   1 2 3 4 5 6 7 8 9 10
Exertion   1 2 3 4 5 6 7 8 9 10
Energy Level   1 2 3 4 5 6 7 8 9 10

Glasses of Water

Breakfast   CALORIES
_____
_____
_____
_____
_____
_____
_____
_____

Lunch   CALORIES
_____
_____
_____
_____
_____
_____
_____

Dinner   CALORIES
_____
_____
_____
_____
_____
_____
_____

W O D
workout of the day

__Warmup__ _____

__Workout__ _____
_____
_____
_____
_____

__Recovery__ _____

Daily Log

| Mon | Tue | Wed | Thur | Fri | Sat | Sun |

S l e e p   1 2 3 4 5 6 7 8 9 10

S t r e s s   1 2 3 4 5 6 7 8 9 10

E x e r t i o n   1 2 3 4 5 6 7 8 9 10

Energy Level   1 2 3 4 5 6 7 8 9 10

Glasses of Water

Breakfast CALORIES

_____

_____

_____

_____

_____

_____

_____

_____

Lunch CALORIES

_____

_____

_____

_____

_____

_____

Dinner CALORIES

_____

_____

_____

_____

_____

_____

W O D
workout of the day

Warmup _____

Workout _____

_____

_____

_____

_____

Recovery _____

Mon   Tue   Wed   Thur   Fri   Sat   Sun

Sleep	1 2 3 4 5 6 7 8 9 10
Stress	1 2 3 4 5 6 7 8 9 10
Exertion	1 2 3 4 5 6 7 8 9 10
Energy Level	1 2 3 4 5 6 7 8 9 10

Glasses of Water

Breakfast   CALORIES

Lunch   CALORIES

Dinner   CALORIES

W O D
workout of the day

Warmup

Workout

Recovery

Month	Day			Daily Log		
Mon	**Tue**	**Wed**	**Thur**	**Fri**	**Sat**	**Sun**

Sleep   1 2 3 4 5 6 7 8 9 10

Stress   1 2 3 4 5 6 7 8 9 10

Exertion   1 2 3 4 5 6 7 8 9 10

Energy Level   1 2 3 4 5 6 7 8 9 10

Glasses of Water

Breakfast CALORIES

Lunch CALORIES

Dinner CALORIES

W O D
workout of the day

Warmup

Workout

Recovery

| Mon | Tue | Wed | Thur | Fri | Sat | Sun |

Sleep   1 2 3 4 5 6 7 8 9 10

Stress   1 2 3 4 5 6 7 8 9 10

Exertion 1 2 3 4 5 6 7 8 9 10

Energy Level 1 2 3 4 5 6 7 8 9 10

Glasses of Water

Breakfast   CALORIES

_____

_____

_____

_____

_____

_____

Lunch   CALORIES

_____

_____

_____

_____

_____

_____

Dinner   CALORIES

_____

_____

_____

_____

_____

_____

W O D
workout of the day

Warmup _____

Workout _____

_____

_____

_____

_____

Recovery _____

Mon	Tue	Wed	Thur	Fri	Sat	Sun

Sleep   1 2 3 4 5 6 7 8 9 10

Stress   1 2 3 4 5 6 7 8 9 10

Exertion   1 2 3 4 5 6 7 8 9 10

Energy Level   1 2 3 4 5 6 7 8 9 10

Glasses of Water

Breakfast   CALORIES

Lunch   CALORIES

Dinner   CALORIES

W O D
workout of the day

Warmup

Workout

Recovery

| Mon | Tue | Wed | Thur | Fri | Sat | Sun |

Sleep   1 2 3 4 5 6 7 8 9 10
Stress   1 2 3 4 5 6 7 8 9 10
Exertion   1 2 3 4 5 6 7 8 9 10
Energy Level   1 2 3 4 5 6 7 8 9 10

Glasses of Water

Breakfast   CALORIES

_____
_____
_____
_____
_____
_____
_____

Lunch   CALORIES

_____
_____
_____
_____
_____
_____

Dinner   CALORIES

_____
_____
_____
_____
_____
_____

W O D
workout of the day

Warmup _____

Workout _____
_____
_____
_____
_____
_____

Recovery _____

Month	Day		Daily Log

Mon	Tue	Wed	Thur	Fri	Sat	Sun

Sleep 1 2 3 4 5 6 7 8 9 10

Stress 1 2 3 4 5 6 7 8 9 10

Exertion 1 2 3 4 5 6 7 8 9 10

Energy Level 1 2 3 4 5 6 7 8 9 10

Glasses of Water

Breakfast CALORIES

_____

_____

_____

_____

_____

_____

_____

_____

Lunch CALORIES

_____

_____

_____

_____

_____

_____

_____

Dinner CALORIES

_____

_____

_____

_____

_____

_____

_____

W O D
workout of the day

Warmup _____

Workout _____

_____

_____

_____

_____

Recovery _____

Mon   Tue   Wed   Thur   Fri   Sat   Sun

Sleep   1 2 3 4 5 6 7 8 9 10   Breakfast   CALORIE
Stress   1 2 3 4 5 6 7 8 9 10
Exertion   1 2 3 4 5 6 7 8 9 10   _____
Energy Level   1 2 3 4 5 6 7 8 9 10   _____

Glasses of Water

_____

_____

_____

_____

_____

Lunch	CALORIES		Dinner	CALORIES
_____			_____	
_____			_____	
_____			_____	
_____			_____	
_____			_____	
_____			_____	

W   O   D
workout of the day

Warmup   _____

Workout _____

_____

_____

_____

_____

Recovery _____

Month	Day			Daily Log

Mon	Tue	Wed	Thur	Fri	Sat	Sun

S l e e p   1 2 3 4 5 6 7 8 9 10

S t r e s s   1 2 3 4 5 6 7 8 9 10

Exertion   1 2 3 4 5 6 7 8 9 10

Energy Level   1 2 3 4 5 6 7 8 9 10

Glasses of Water

Breakfast — CALORIES

Lunch — CALORIES

Dinner — CALORIES

W O D
workout of the day

Warmup

Workout

Recovery

| Month | | Day | | | | | |

Mon	Tue	Wed	Thur	Fri	Sat	Sun

Sleep   1 2 3 4 5 6 7 8 9 10
Stress   1 2 3 4 5 6 7 8 9 10
Exertion   1 2 3 4 5 6 7 8 9 10
Energy Level 1 2 3 4 5 6 7 8 9 10

Glasses of Water

Breakfast   CALORIE

_____
_____
_____
_____
_____
_____
_____

Lunch   CALORIES

_____
_____
_____
_____
_____
_____

Dinner   CALORIE

_____
_____
_____
_____
_____
_____

W O D
workout of the day

Warmup _____

Workout _____

_____
_____
_____

Recovery _____

| Mon | Tue | Wed | Thur | Fri | Sat | Sun |

Sleep 1 2 3 4 5 6 7 8 9 10

Stress 1 2 3 4 5 6 7 8 9 10

Exertion 1 2 3 4 5 6 7 8 9 10

Energy Level 1 2 3 4 5 6 7 8 9 10

Glasses of Water

Breakfast CALORIES

_____

_____

_____

_____

_____

_____

_____

_____

Lunch CALORIES

_____
_____
_____
_____
_____
_____
_____

Dinner CALORIES

_____
_____
_____
_____
_____
_____
_____

W O D
workout of the day

Warmup _____

Workout _____

_____
_____
_____
_____
_____

Recovery _____

Mon   Tue   Wed   Thur   Fri   Sat   Sun

Sleep	1 2 3 4 5 6 7 8 9 10	Breakfast	CALORIE
Stress	1 2 3 4 5 6 7 8 9 10		
Exertion	1 2 3 4 5 6 7 8 9 10		
Energy Level	1 2 3 4 5 6 7 8 9 10		

Glasses of Water

Lunch	CALORIES	Dinner	CALORIE

W O D
workout of the day

Warmup

Workout

Recovery

Mon	Tue	Wed	Thur	Fri	Sat	Sun

Sleep   1 2 3 4 5 6 7 8 9 10
Stress   1 2 3 4 5 6 7 8 9 10
Exertion   1 2 3 4 5 6 7 8 9 10
Energy Level 1 2 3 4 5 6 7 8 9 10

Glasses of Water

Breakfast   CALORIES

_____

_____

_____

_____

_____

_____

_____

Lunch   CALORIES

_____

_____

_____

_____

_____

_____

Dinner   CALORIES

_____

_____

_____

_____

_____

_____

_____

W O D
workout of the day

Warmup _____

Workout _____

_____

_____

_____

_____

Recovery _____

Month	Day				Daily Log	

Mon	Tue	Wed	Thur	Fri	Sat	Sun

Sleep   1 2 3 4 5 6 7 8 9 10

Stress   1 2 3 4 5 6 7 8 9 10

Exertion   1 2 3 4 5 6 7 8 9 10

Energy Level   1 2 3 4 5 6 7 8 9 10

Breakfast   CALORIE

Glasses of Water

Lunch   CALORIES

Dinner   CALORIE

W O D
workout of the day

Warmup

Workout

Recovery

CPSIA information can be obtained
at www.ICGtesting.com
Printed in the USA
LVHW050754281018
595066LV00004B/31/P